# STUART HOFFMAN

# GYM MOTIVATION

## *TOP 5 WAYS TO STAY MOTIVATED AT THE GYM*

First edition

This book was professionally typeset on Reedsy.
Find out more at reedsy.com

# Contents

# 1

# Introduction

Whether you're thinking about starting your fitness journey or have already begun your journey, this book is here to help you navigate through your valleys and break through your plateaus. Fitness journeys are rough, there is no easy way to say that. If someone tells you otherwise, run the other way!

My name is Stuart Hoffman and I wanted to share with you my journey and 5 ways to help you stay motivated during your journey and going to the gym. The gym can be a scary place. There are lots of machines that have instructions on them letting you know how to use the machine. Let's be honest though, most of them don't even make sense in the way the machine was designed and the illustration that is provided. Nobody wants to be "That" individual that is caught not using the machine correctly and will be recorded only to be made fun of on someone else's social media account for likes and follows. I am not a personal trainer nor a certified health expert in any way. What I am is an experienced individual who was once in your shoes. Someone setting out on a journey to change their life, to push themselves to achieve goals that have never been achieved yet. We will dive into this more in Chapter

1 "Find your reason", but you must have a reason as to why you want that specific goal. This is why most people give up, their reason why, is not strong enough, or that they really don't want it. They are tricking themselves into believing they want or need it.

The 5 ways to help you stay motivated during your journey at the gym that I am about to share with you resonates deeply with me because these are what really helped me during my low points where all I wanted to do was give up and throw in the towel. I hope you find these reasons as impactful and provide you with the strength you need to achieve your goals. If you can master these steps, not only will it help you in your fitness journey, but it will also be able to provide you with valuable insights and skills that transfer over into your daily lives, making you a better version of yourself.

Enjoy!

2

# Chapter 1: Find your reason

*"When you walk in purpose, you collide with destiny."-Ralph Buchanan-*

Before you can begin your fitness journey, you must, "find your reason". There are many reasons to choose from. It could be that you're overweight and you rely on the assistance of others to help or take care of you, or the simple fact that you know you're at risk of heart disease, type 2 diabetes, high blood pressure, cancer, and other chronic conditions. Sometimes the knowledge of simple health issues that you're exposing yourself to is enough to change. You might have kids, or want kids. Don't you want to be around when they are growing up? Don't you want to be a part of their life? Not only be a part of their life, but have an impact on them and help develop them into our next generation? Time goes fast! Before we know it, our kids are all grown up and moving on. I used to work at a job where I was putting in so much overtime I was missing out on key milestones in my kids' life. I told myself I am working lots of hours so that I can provide a good life for them and give them everything they want. One of my biggest regrets is not being around and cherishing those memories and milestones of my kids growing up. Even though I was working and not around, your physical health can sometimes cause you to be absent because you can't go and do the things your kids want to do.Don't make the same mistake I did. It was an expensive one and It's something I can never get back.

Additional reasons might be performance based. Maybe you're a high school athlete, college athlete, or professional athlete. Maybe you're an avid runner preparing for a marathon, or a cyclist preparing for a race. You also might be trying to achieve a specific aesthetic look, or want to compete in a bodybuilding competition. Whatever you are doing, you must define your reason as to why you want to achieve what you're about to embark on. This will be a lighthouse guiding your ship away from the shallows on stormy days. I would be lying to you if I told you this process would be an easy one. It's not going to be. You will have your highs and your lows. That's just how it is. You will not be able to enjoy the highs without the lows either. So along your journey, take time to think and reflect where you are at. Are you experiencing a high? Or are you experiencing a low? And reflect on where you're at. This will help you along your journey and allow you to understand what changes (big or small) you need to make in order to get back on track or stay on track. Taking the time to reflect will build a profound characteristic that will carry over into daily life. This characteristic is "self awareness". Self awareness is: *"an awareness of one's own personality or individuality"*. When we are self aware, we can clearly define our personalities and habits that are beneficial and help us, and that have a negative impact on us. When we can clearly identify our weaknesses and what is holding us back we can make the necessary adjustments in our lives to help us achieve our goals. This is and will forever be an ongoing process. Throughout your journey, you will develop new habits that are good, and others that are detrimental to your goals. Another reason to always take time and reflect on you and where you are in your journey and make the necessary changes.

You might be an individual whose reason might simply be proving to yourself that you can set and achieve hard goals. If you're someone who has never set a goal, or someone who has never completed goals. The gym is actually a great place to start. Even if it's just showing up and walking on the treadmill for thirty minutes a day. You can do that! Or you might be after developing characteristics and attributes like Discipline, Consistency, Sacrifice, Self Control, Dedication, etc. Whether you like it or not, the development of these characteristics will just come naturally. So if anything else, it's like a cherry on top, or a free gift, and who doesn't like a free gift, right?

This is what we are after. The "reason" you choose must drive you to want to set and achieve goals in a way to where you can take complete control of your life. You want to be in complete control, that way there are no limiting factors or excuses.

With that said, Take time now and define your reason!

# Chapter 2: Set Goals

*"Setting goals is the first step in turning the invisible into the visible"*
*-Anthony Robbins-*

S etting goals in my opinion is one of the most overlooked and underrated aspects of being able to stay motivated at the gym. Without goals, you have no vision. I want to specifically focus on your "Gym" goals. Not necessarily your overall goals and what you're trying to achieve, but specifically the goals you set for yourself at the gym. One important thing to keep in mind with goals is that if you are not thinking about them consistently, how are you going to be able to work at those goals on a day to day basis? You can not! It will not happen. You need to write down your goals and make them visible to you. Making these goals visible to you will remind yourself daily what you committed yourself to and help remind and motivate you to keep going. Too many times in my life have I made a goal, wrote it down on paper, and put it in a safe place for me to revisit. Do you know how many times I would revisit my goals? Yup, you guessed it. Hardly never. It wasn't until I had racked up over ten thousand dollars worth of credit card debt that I decided to set a goal for myself and my wife to work towards so we could start chipping away at our debt. To put things into perspective, our credit card payments together were well over what we were paying on our monthly mortgage. Crazy to think about. I was basically paying for two homes, but without the benefit of what a second home could have done for us financially. Being fed up and feeling trapped financially, my wife and I created a plan and set goals on how we were going to climb this mountain. It wasn't going to be easy. But we knew we could do it. We wrote down our goals and discussed it several times. This time it was going to be different. We went to the store and bought a very large white board and hung it up in our bathroom. We then proceeded to list off all the items we owned money on along with the monthly payment and interest rate of each. Every month we would go through and update all our numbers. Little by little, we were able to start eliminating all these line items one by one until they were all gone. I am fairly certain that this would not have happened if my wife and I did not write down these goals and our plan to achieve them and place it strategically in a position that both in the morning and evening we were able to see all the numbers and remember what we were trying to accomplish.

I like to break my goals down into two main categories. Main goals and Sub goals. My main goals are more like milestone benchmarks and what I am working towards. These goals should seem and feel at first glance like they are more on the unachievable side. However, as we put our heads down and get to work, little by little we will chip away at this goal until we accomplish it. How do you climb a mountain? Little by little, right? One foot in front of the other. Back squatting two hundred and twenty five pounds might seem like a crazy goal for someone jumping into weightlifting for the first time. However, every week we progressively get stronger and stronger until we can get that weight for one repetition. Then the next week we build to that same weight for two repetitions. Before you know it, you will be repping that weight for a warm up set. We may have had a setback or two along the way, tweaked a back and had to take time off to recover, but just like one foot in front of the other, you worked your way back to where you were and exceeded your goal. Again, I want to reiterate the importance of your goals, and make sure that they are in the forefront of your mind. Even if you have to write your goals on a three x five note card and say them out loud before you enter the gym while you're sitting in your car. Whatever you need to do, you have to see these goals daily.

My sub goals are all the smaller goals I will need to accomplish to hit those main goals or milestones. You have to start somewhere right? Start small, there is no such thing as a small and useless goal. Believe it or not, but simply setting simple goals at the gym that get you moving and in the right direction has a waterfall effect on all your other goals and aspirations. It becomes easier to achieve goals when you start to get a little momentum on your side, and the gym is an easy way to start to build your momentum. Stacking small wins will motivate you to continue and keep going. It's like waking up every morning and making your bed. It's such an easy task to do, but it's a "W" in the win/lose column. When you start stacking your wins throughout the day, you win the day. When you stack your days with wins, you win the week. When you stack your weeks with wins, you win the month. And when you stack your months with wins, you win the year! It's a simple concept but a very powerful one. Take a boulder for example, if it starts to roll and you step in front immediately to stop it, it's pretty easy to stop right? But if that same boulder has a head start and it builds momentum, it becomes impossible to stop. Goal setting and achieving is very similar. You will start small on your goals, and as you progress through the journey, you will start to gain momentum and crush all the other goals that are placed in the way. The coolest part about all this is that the momentum will continue with you throughout the day, helping you stay focused on all the tasks at hand and give you the confidence to complete all the tasks needed that day either at work or at home. Momentum is key!

4

# Chapter 3: Track your progress

"Once you start tracking your goals, you're able to see the small, day by day<br>
progress that you might not otherwise notice"<br>
-Betsy Tamser Jaime-

There are several ways to track your progress through your journey. I'll touch briefly on a few that have helped me out tremendously throughout my journey in hopes it will help you. Never get down on yourself when your numbers fluctuate. Throughout your journey, your measurements will not always go in the direction you are hoping for. So if we can go into this journey understanding this simple concept, we will be able to push through and get consistent with our tracking. Do not get discouraged, this is part of the process! Ultimately, we are making steps in the right direction, and that is what matters.

**Journals** - YES! These are still a thing! YES, I am talking about a good ole journal with pen and/or paper. Obviously, you're going to want to write down the exercise of your choice. Be very specific! How much weight, how many repetitions, how many sets and the date. Same thing would apply if you were running. How long did it take you to run 2 miles, what was your pace, was it at an incline? Ect. This is important because the next time you do the same workout, you have something to look back on as a reference. This will also give you the confidence you need to continue to push yourself in weight, repetitions, and sets. There have been countless times where I forget what I have already achieved, so I end up doing the same thing. If I am doing the same workout week after week, without progressing in any area, how can I expect to get bigger, faster, or stronger? I can't! So write it down and revisit it multiple times. Continue to push yourself on every workout. Make your vision clear and workout with a purpose, don't just show up and run through the movements. When you do this, this is not a formula of success, nor is it retainable. This is probably one of the reasons why most people give up at the gym. The monotonous routines that get boring and are longer fun or challenging for you. Do not be afraid to incorporate new movements and workouts as this will help keep your workouts different, fun, and exciting. Be safe! Increasing weight is a privilege. Make sure you have proper form before increasing weight. Push yourself into doing new and uncomfortable things. You need to get comfortable being uncomfortable. This is another great characteristic that will carry over in all you do.

**Measurements** - This one is pretty self explanatory. You will want to make note of your body measurements. Run a small tape measure around your arms, shoulders, chest, stomach, hips, thighs, and calves. Or wherever you want to keep track. This is totally up to you. I would pick a time that is that works for you and that you can make a consistent habit out of it. Again, consistency is the name of the game. If you can be consistent at something, your ability to be successful dramatically increases. Find a time that works for you, and stick to that. If you would prefer the evening that's fine too. What we don't want is that sometimes you take your measurements in the morning and other days you do it midday or evenings. When you do that you have to factor in all the other variables that will play into the results you're getting. For me, I would measure myself in the mornings after my workouts.  I figured this would be the best time for me to do it so that I could get an accurate weight along with my measurements. Personally, I like to work out first thing in the morning on an empty stomach (in most cases). I do my measurements in the morning because this is normally when I am at my lightest (my true weight).  I am not fighting any potential bloating around my stomach that could affect my measurement numbers. Taking measurements in the morning allowed me to remove most of the variables so I could get as accurate and consistent numbers as I could with where my body is at.

**Photos** - This is something that most people overlook. I never really liked taking pictures along my journey because I never really liked the way I looked.  It embarrassed me. Week after week, month after month your body can play mind tricks on you to trick you into thinking you're not making progress. The power that taking photos has is when you gather enough photo information, you can pull up the two photos side by side and compare the two.  As disgusted as you feel in the moment taking photos of yourself, there is an immense amount of joy when you pull up the comparison and can actually see the muffin top disappearing, or the thigh gap appearing. Not only does it bring you a sense of accomplishment, but it also affirms that what you are doing is working. You can always refer back to your photo library when you are struggling. Use this as motivation because you will need to. I have needed to go back several times just to compare where I am at versus when I started. Everytime I have done it, it has provided a nice little kick in the pants to keep going. I still go back to this date and review these photos when I am having a difficult time with my diet, or just struggling in general. It's hard to compare weight loss from week to week with photos. But if you use them from month to month, now that is powerful! Again, get consistent with this. Whatever you need to do, do it. Create a secure folder on your phone and store all those photos in there if you want. Just start collecting the data. You will be surprised how much strength this will give you when you are struggling. Don't believe me, try it! I dare you!

**Apps** - We live in a really exciting time where we have a lot of apps out there that can help with tracking our progress. You don't have to download these apps. I just wanted to mention a tool and resource that you could use. Recently I have been using an app that holds all my measurements and photos together. The app will allow me to pull up the two photos side by side to compare. It will also show me all the measurements with the photo, so I can see in what direction I am trending. Again, you might feel like you want to keep all this information private and in a secure location. Do what will ultimately make you feel good about yourself. If you like the old school way of just writing things down on paper and then have your photos saved on your phone, you can do that. One thing I love about the whole fitness journey is that there are multiple ways that you can succeed at this. Part of your success will be implementing everything we have talked about, and are going to talk about in your life and your lifestyle. The end result may be the same, but there are many paths to achieve it. So pick a path that works for you and only you. You got this!

**Scans** - What I am referring to here is body scans, or DEXA scans. This might be the most powerful tool, in my opinion, to help you along your journey to staying motivated at the gym in tracking your progress. The scan will be able to tell you everything else that the scale, photos, and measurements can't. DEXA stands for dual energy x-ray absorptiometry. I know a mouthful right? And how does this relate to weight loss, or being able to track your progress. Let me tell you. The scan will calculate (more accurately) how much body fat you have. It will also calculate how much muscle mass and your bone density. If you're trying to lose weight, and only using a scale, you could become very discouraged that the scale is maintaining your current weight, or you could be going up in weight. But what you're not realizing is that you could be losing body fat, and putting on muscle. Muscle weighs more than fat, so from a scale/weight standpoint you could be misled to believe you're putting fat on when in reality this is far from the case. You could be an athlete looking to bulk and put on weight. Again, you might see the scale increasing because you're bulking, but ask yourself, the weight you're putting on, is it good weight or bad weight? Is the weight in the form of muscle? Or fat? This is exactly why you need to get these scans done. We need all the information so we can understand what is actually happening to our body when we see and track our measurements. So how much does this scan cost? It sounds expensive right? Well if you had money to spend, I would say go spend it on the most accurate one you have in your area. But, if you're like me, and don't want or have money to spend on imaging, then there are very good and accurate scans available to do for a minimal cost or even free. I have a local supplement shop in my area that has an accurate scanner that will allow anyone to scan for under $50 bucks. However, if you buy supplements there from them, then you can scan for free. I would say check your area and see what's available for you. Can I just buy a body fat scale from like amazon? The answer is yes, however *"they have been proven to not be very accurate due to the testing being on a small number of people"* Said Dr. Woolcott. *"The scales underestimate or overestimate body fat percentages by quite a lot"*. My general rule of thumb is use the numbers just to track if I am trending in the right direction or not between my DEXA scans. I have one of those weight loss scales that tracks body fat, and I can say that my DEXA body scans have been more accurate. There have been times where my DEXA scan will say I am 16%-18% body fat while my at home scanner will say I have over 25%. 16% or even 18% sounds so much better than 25%. That's a huge difference, and something as small as that could be the difference between giving up and continuing to push forward.

I hope you enjoyed my insight as to what and why you should be tracking on a weekly basis. I can't express enough that you have to find what works for you and just be consistent at it. If you are feeling overwhelmed a bit, like that's a lot. It's OK. Just pick a few and implement them today! If you do, I can promise this will have a direct impact on your vision and goals moving forward.

5

# Chapter 4: Endure the process

*"There is no royal road to anything, one thing at a time, all things in succession. That which grows fast, withers as rapidly. That which grows slowly, endures.*
*-Josiah Gilbert Holland-*

I love this quote. This resonates with me so much and I hope it resonates with you as well. Anything that is easy will diminish just as fast. I think of all those videos, and I know you have seen them that solicit losing weight fast, and getting in the best shape of your life quickly. While lots of these videos or ads provide a lot of valuable and true information, true transformation takes time. I am sorry, but it is what it is and there is no sugar coating that.I mean think about it. If you are overweight, you didn't just wake up one day overweight. It took a while, even years of developing bad habits and nutrition to put on all that excess weight. So in order to get back, or get somewhere you have never been, it's a process, a journey, and it will take time. It should take time, because along the way you are developing the right mindset, characteristics, and disciplines necessary to be a better and more successful you. The longer it takes the more valuable it will

16

become to you. One definition of endurance is *"the ability or strength to continue or last, especially despite fatigue, stress, or other adverse conditions."* Part of my success has been accepting that this change will take time. This has literally been the foundation of my success in my journey. Just like a home needs a solid foundation in order to stay standing, you will need a solid foundation along your journey. You will have very high highs and extremely low lows. It's during the low times that the true character of one shines. Who will you be? Will you be the one that gives up and caves in? Or will you stay strong and endure the journey? I hope I am painting this picture right for you. If you know and understand that you will face some really hard times ahead, this will soften the blow a little bit. If someone gave you a blueprint to become extremely wealthy, and along the way they said you will go through droughts where you wont have very much money, but if you stick to it, you will break through and become wealthy, would you do it? We all would! Why do we treat our fitness journey any differently? We shouldn't. We should learn to embrace the suck and face our challenges head on. What would our lives be if we didn't face challenges? Would it be a life worth living for? We need to learn and adapt, that is how we become our best selves.

One other thing that has helped me dramatically endure the process has been accountability partners and all the individuals I have met at the gym and along the way. An alcoholic has a better chance of abstinence going to AA meetings than doing any other method. Why is that? Keight Humphreys, PhD professor of psychiatry and behavioral science said *"AA works because it's based on social interaction, nothing that members give one another emotional support as well as practical tips to refrain from drinking. If you want to change your behavior, find some other people who are trying to make the same change."* Having people that share the same goals and visions you have is motivating in itself. Knowing that other people are putting work in will help you. Opening up and talking with people at the gym and outside the gym will help. You will be able to establish friendships and trust. Opening up to them about your journey will also allow you to be vulnerable and open to suggestions, especially if they are further along in the process then you are. I am sure you have heard that if you want to become wealthy, then surround yourself with wealthy people. Why is that? Because there is lots to learn from them. I recently completed a program designed around fathers who wanted to take control of their lives again. Within that program, I met people I have never met before. Our only interaction was through the app and video calls. I watched a video of one other student who was doing his accountability portion. After watching his video, I wanted to reach out personally to him. We exchanged numbers and continue to chat on a regular basis. We both completed this course over 3 years ago now. Even though we have never met in person before, we still use this valuable tool to keep each other accountable for our goals and aspirations. We absolutely love it! Another amazing point to this would be that _YOU_ get to play a significant role in someone else's life. You could be the reason why they were successful. If that doesn't get you going, I don't know what else would.

6

# Chapter 5: Love your results

*"Our greatest weakness lies in giving up. The most certain way to succeed is always to try just one more time"*
*-Thomas Eddison-*

We had to save the best for last. This is probably the hardest thing you might face. Love your results. Big or small. Celebrate your achievements. No I am not saying to go and binge eat your favorite meals or take a week off of your program. But be proud and make sure you celebrate your wins. When you can learn to love and appreciate your accomplishments, it invites positive thinking and self worth into your life. Ask yourself, if you were to improve in positive thinking and self worth in your life right now, would your life get any better? I know mine would. Too many times we get caught up in the negativity that surrounds us on a daily basis. This, believe it or not, has a negative impact on our lives. You are and always will be your worst critic. Do not let yourself tear yourself down and convince yourself that you are incapable of making a change in your life.

As you start to celebrate the wins in your life, you will start to recognize a burning desire to keep going. Not only will you be able to keep going, but now you will be able to be a well of accomplishments that others can rely on from time to time from you.  If there is one thing that really, truly brings a lot of happiness, it's being able to serve and help others. If you have not experienced that yet, I encourage you to look for opportunities to serve and uplift others around you. Watching others succeed and achieve their goals because you played an immense role in that is unexplainable. Success is contagious, once you experience a little bit, you crave more. This is probably one of the few things where it's OK or even suggested that you over indulge.

# 7

# Conclusion

Wherever you are at in your journey, I hope these steps will help you in some way or another. Maybe you are already doing all these things, or maybe you're already doing a few. Remember that there is always room for improvement though. So if you're already doing some of these things, start to develop the other skills necessary to help you stay on track so you can achieve your vision and become the best version of yourself.

The only thing stopping you is you. Do not give up. Keep going! Failure only is present when you give up. As long as you keep going, no matter how many times you fall or stumble, get up! One step at a time. One foot in front of the other. Enjoy the journey. It's not a sprint, this is a marathon. Pace yourself and go at your own speed. The gym is a starting point for a whole new and approved you. We discussed several times how we can improve ourselves and develop better attributes and characteristics to become better individuals. These characteristics and attributes will carry over into your jobs, relationships, and family. Now it's your turn.

Get after it!

www.ingramcontent.com/pod-product-compliance
Lightning Source LLC
Chambersburg PA
CBHW060911260726

48661CB00008B/3587